Dukan Diet Attack Phase

Recipes and Diet Plan for the Dukan Diet Phase 1

Table of Contents

Introduction

The Dukan Diet was conceptualized in 2000 by a French nutritionist and general practitioner named Pierre Dukan. The promise behind the Dukan Diet is a permanent weight loss of 10 pounds within the first week of embarking on the diet—with the provision that you follow the Dukan Diet Rules.

In the heart of the Dukan Diet rule is a daily 20-minute walk and consumption of water, oat bran and lean protein. The driving principle behind the diet is that if you limit your carbohydrate intake, you are forcing your body to burn fat.

In the Dukan Diet you are allowed to eat as much food as you want, provided that these foods belong to the list of foods okayed by the diet—which of course only allows a handful few of carbs. All in all the Dukan Diet lists a hundred of allowed foods in the diet, 28 of which is plant based and the rest comes from animal sources.

Chapter 1: The Different Phases of the Dukan Diet

The Dukan Diet is composed of four different phases that they need to go through and each phase is different from the other.

First Phase: Attack Phase

The attack phase is basically the part where the dieter kick starts their metabolism by consuming only protein foods within a span of one to seven days. It is aimed that within two days of starting the Attack Phase, dieters can experience rapid weight loss. By the end of the attack phase, as much as 4.4 to 6.6 pounds is lost.

Since this book is all about the Dukan Diet's Attack phase, you will learn more about this phase in later subheadings. First, let's just settle for a short description of phases to get a good overview of the diet.

Second Phase: Cruise Phase

The cruise phase is the second phase of the Dukan Diet and it can last for several months—which depend on the dieters' targeted weight. In this phase, the weight loss tapers down to 1 pound per week. So if you need to lose 20 pounds more (aside from the weight lost from the Attack Phase) then you would need to stick to the Cruise Phase for 20 weeks or until such time that you reach your desired weight.

During this phase, fruits are not allowed in the diet, but there is an addition of 28 specific veggies. This helps dieters to lose weight gradually.

Third Phase: Consolidation Phase

The consolidation phase is the third phase of the Dukan Diet and it lasts depending on how much weight you have lost. So, for each pound you have lost since you started the Dukan Diet, multiply that to five days and that's the total length of the consolidation phase.

During this phase, the dieter is urged to choose a specific day of the week to stick to a core diet of protein. So if you choose Saturday, this means that for the whole duration of the consolidation phase, you are designating Saturdays as your day of eating only protein.

In the consolidation phase, you are allowed to eat unlimited quantities of vegetables and protein. You are also allowed to have at least one to two servings of starchy food. Also, in a week you will be able to have two celebration MEALS (not day, okay?) In a celebration meal, you can eat whatever you like to eat and whatever quantity—of course prudence also plays an important role here folks.

Phase Four: Stabilization Phase

The last phase of the Dukan Diet, which is known as the Stabilization Phase is the maintenance part of the diet. At this point, you already have your desired weight and you are just maintaining the said weight.

There's only a few guiding rules during the fourth phase of the Dukan Diet and these are:

- Do a 20-minute walk or exercise daily.
- Eat 3 tbsps of oat bran each day.

- Designate one day in a week for your "Just Protein Day" this means that you are not going to eat anything but protein.

Chapter 2: Getting to Know Dukan Diet's Attack Phase

As we have mentioned earlier, the first step to the Dukan Diet is the Attack Phase which is also known as the Protein Phase, wherein dieters are urged to eat meat or protein only for a rapid weight loss. This is an important feature of the diet because the sudden drop of weight easily motivates people to stick to the diet. The phase takes between one to seven days to complete and weight loss can be seen by day two.

Although there is carbohydrate included in the Attack Phase, but this is only 1 ½ tbsps of oat bran a day. So, why is oat bran included in the Attack Phase? It has been found that oat bran contains a huge amount of fiber and can increase in size inside the stomach up to 20 times. This means that it can help suppress appetite. Further, oat bran's fibrous carbohydrates are not easily digested by the stomach and are just flushed away from the body without being metabolized—so it doesn't end up in your fatty tissues. And during the attack phase, you are encouraged to drink as much as 1.5 liters of water a day.

Important Information about the Attack Phase

Before you start the Dukan Diet Attack Phase, here is a complete list of important notes about the diet to help you get started.

How Long Does Attack Phase Last?

The attack phase lasts between one to seven days and actually depends on how much weight you need to lose. See below for guidelines on how many days you should be in the attack phase:

- If you need to lose more than 40 pounds of weight, then you have to undergo the attack phase for seven days. Do consult with your physician before starting on the diet so that you will be advised properly.
- If you need to lose 15 to 30 pounds of weight, then you need to undergo the attack phase for three to five days.
- If you need to lose 10 pounds or less, then undergo the Attack phase for one or two days.

What Are The Foods That I Can Eat?

Here is a complete list of the foods that you can eat during the Attack phase. Unless otherwise stipulated below, the meat that you should eat should be less than 5% fat.

- 2% fat or low fat dairy products – fat free milk, plain yogurt or fat free quark, fat free Greek yogurt, fat free fromage frais and fat free cottage cheese.
- Only two eggs per day, but you can have unlimited egg whites. If you have high cholesterol, watch for the egg yolks. Hen's or quail eggs are highly desired.
- Crustaceans and shellfish – whelks, shrimps, scallops, prawns, oysters, mussels, gambas or Mediterranean prawns, lobster, Dublin bay prawns, crayfish or crawfish, crab, cockles, clams, and squid.
- Any kind and type of fish except those that have sauces or are canned in oil – mullet, herring, salmon, fish roe and whiting from cod, turbot, tuna, swordfish, skate, sea bream, sardines, smoked salmon, salmon, red mullet, salmon trout or rainbow trout, coley or Pollock, plaice, monkfish, mackerel, herring,

halibut, hake, haddock, Grey mullet, Dover sole, lemon or dab sole, surimi or crabsticks, cod, and bass.
- Chicken liver, veal and beef
- Lean and low fat ham
- Turkey and chicken except for the skin – turkey, quail, ostrich, guinea fowl, poussin, and chicken.
- Rabbit, veal or lean beef—minced meat should be less than 10% fat and avoid ribs.
- Sugar free chewing gum, sugar free natural ketchup in moderation, lemon juice as spice and not for drinking, onion as spice, garlic, herbs, spices, mustard, vinegar and sweeteners that are not fructose based.
- Tofu

Any Side Effects That I should Know of During the Attack Phase?

When you go through the Attack Phase, the diet is filled with protein food sources. Since, you are feeding your body with protein as the fuel source, the body goes into ketosis—which simply means that your body is digesting the proteins to fuel the body's energy needs and produces ketones as byproducts which are then eliminated via the urine. This is the reason behind why you are urged to drink plenty of water while on a Dukan Diet.

Further, you may also experience dry mouth and bad breath which is related to ketosis. Again, if you drink plenty of water, this undesired effect can easily be prevented. You can likewise chew a sugar free gum to prevent episodes of bad breath.

Another side effect of the diet is constipation which is a common side effect of a diet rich in protein. This problem is easily solved with drinking a lot of water plus the inclusion of oat bran in your diet. So all in all, the Dukan Diet is a safe way to lose weight.

Diet Tips for the Attack Phase

So, here are some helpful tips to aid you in the first phase of the Dukan Diet. You have to know that changing your diet is not as easy as it sounds, therefor be aware that during the first few days of the diet, it will be a bit hard because you would need to fight off your old eating habits plus your addiction to foods like chocolate and other sugars. But, here are some tips to help you during the Attack Phase of the Dukan Diet:

- Ensure that you eat at least 3 meals a day with a good sized portion to ensure that you won't go hungry until your next meal because in this diet, hunger is your number one enemy which can easily push you to eat carbs.
- During the first days of the Attack phase, it is common to feel easily exhausted and feel a bit tired since your body is still adjusting to your new diet. So, I advise you to not include strenuous activities or exercises during the first few days of your diet. The carb cravings and tiredness goes away after three days and after that, a lot of dieters have reported that they became more energetic.
- Further, during the first few days of the diet, this is when you will feel the side effects of constipation due to the pure protein diet. That's why you are urged to drink plenty of water. Plus eating the required amount of oat bran daily also helps in adding fiber to your diet to prevent constipation.
- If during the first five days of undergoing the Attack Phase you do not see any improvement in weight, you need to go to the next phase which is the cruise phase. This is true even if you have planned your attack phase a few days longer.

Chapter 3: Dukan Diet Attack Phase Meal Recipes

In this chapter, I have provided you with a complete 7-day meal plan recipes. I hope you will enjoy creating these dishes towards a new you. The recipes that I have made for you below do not include serving sizes since in the Dukan Diet's Attack Phase you do not have limited portions—in fact you can eat a limitless amount of protein. Also, I encourage you to take the oat bran early in the morning along with your breakfast. Some of the breakfast meals though already contain oat bran, if this is so, no need to add oat bran to your diet for the day.

7-Day Meal Plan Menu

Breakfast	
Monday	Dukan Diet Toast from Oat Bran (eat only ½ of recipe) Ham
Tuesday	Herbed Omelet On Oat Bran Toast
Wednesday	Oat Bran Porridge with Vanilla (eat only ½ of recipe)

	Zero Fat Milk
Thursday	Pan Fried Trout
Friday	Dukan Diet Pancake with Oat Bran
Saturday	Grilled Halibut
Sunday	Oat Bran Cinnamon Pancake

Lunch	
Monday	Cocktail Of Prawns
Tuesday	Baked Salmon
Wednesday	Vietnamese Beef
Thursday	Turkey Burger Cajun Style
Friday	Sea-food Spanish Style
Saturday	Grilled Cod
Sunday	Baked Mussels

Snack	
Monday	Oat Bran Muffin
Tuesday	Meringue
Wednesday	Oat Bran Cookies (eat no more than 2 pcs in a day)
Thursday	Ginger and Oat Bran Biscuits
Friday	Cappuccino Flavored Dukan Frappe
Saturday	Fro-Yo
Sunday	Cheese-cake Cupcakes

Dinner	
Monday	Grilled Lamb Chops
Tuesday	Beef Kebabs
Wednesday	Chicken Curry
Thursday	Meat Loaf
Friday	Tofu Stir Fry
Saturday	Lamb Rack
Sunday	Tandoori Chicken

Breakfast Recipes

Dukan Diet Toast from Oat Bran

Ingredients:
2 egg whites or 1 egg
2 tbsps of zero fat yogurt
3 tbsps of oat bran

Directions:

1) In a big bowl, beat egg whites or egg in order to add a bit of air.
2) Add and mix thoroughly oat bran and yogurt.
3) On a nonstick small fry pan, grease a bit with cooking spray and cook toast by pouring desired amount on pan and cook like a pan cake. It is good to use egg rings to make perfect a circle.
4) Once one side of the toast is cooked and you have flipped it over, try to press the toast down a bit for around ten counts.
5) Remove from pan and you can enjoy hot or cold. You can also reheat in the microwave or toaster for future use.

Herbed Omelet

Ingredients:
Pepper and salt to taste
1 tbsp chopped green onions
½ tsp dried parsley
½ tsp garlic powder
1 tbsp skim milk
1 egg white
1 whole egg

Directions:

1) In a medium bowl, beat eggs together.
2) Season with garlic powder, parsley, green onions, pepper and salt. Whisk well.
3) Add skim milk and whisk to combine.
4) On medium fire, place a small nonstick skillet and grease with cooking spray.
5) Once heated, pour egg mixture, cover and cook for two to three minutes.
6) With a spatula, flip omelet over and cook for a minute.
7) Remove from fire and enjoy.

Oat Bran Porridge with Vanilla

Ingredients:
1 tbsp Truvia
½ tsp vanilla
125 ml zero fat milk or skim milk
3 tbsps oat bran

Directions:

1) On a small and microwave safe bowl, heat for 45 second the milk and oat bran.
2) Remove from oven, mix and add Truvia and vanilla. Mix well.
3) Let it rest for 3 minutes to allow oat bran to soak in the milk.
4) Pop in the microwave again and cook for another 45 seconds.
5) Serve and enjoy.

Pan Fried Trout

Ingredients:
Pepper and salt to taste
1 bay leaf
1 lemon
1 trout

Directions:

1) Clean trout and season with lemon, salt and pepper.
2) Place bay leaf in the stomach cavity of trout.
3) On medium fire, place a medium nonstick skillet and place trout once heated.
4) Cook for 5 to 8 minutes per side while covered.
5) Once fully cooked, remove from pan and serve.

Dukan Diet Pancake with Oat Bran

Ingredients:
1 tbsp Truvia
1 ½ tbsps zero fat quark
1 ½ tbsps oat bran
1 beaten egg or 2 beaten egg whites

Directions:

1) In a medium bowl beat well together quark, oat bran and egg.
2) Add Truvia and beat well until dissolved and mixed.
3) In a small nonstick fry pan on medium fire greased with cooking spray add batter and cook for 2 to 3 minutes.
4) Turn over pancake, and cook for a minute.
5) Remove from pan, serve and enjoy.

Grilled Halibut

Ingredients:
4-inch thick halibut steak
¼ tsp ground black pepper
¼ tsp salt
¾ tsp dried dill weed
1 ½ tsps dried parsley
1 ½ tsps onion powder
1 tbsp lemon juice

Directions:

1) In a small bowl, mix all ingredients thoroughly except for halibut.
2) In a dish, spread seasoning mixture all over halibut steaks.
3) Place halibut on preheated medium heat grill and grill for 5 to 6 minutes per side.
4) Remove from grill, transfer on serving plate, serve and enjoy.

Cinnamon Flavored Pancake

Ingredients:
½ tbsp Truvia
¼ tsp cinnamon
A dash of nutmeg
A dash of all-spice
1 ½ tbsps fromage frais
1 ½ tbsps oat bran
2 beaten egg whites

Directions:

1) In a small bowl, mix truvia, spices, fromage frais, oat bran and egg.
2) Whisk thoroughly together.
3) On medium fire, place a nonstick small skillet and grease with cooking spray.
4) Once heated, pour battar and cook for 2 to 3 minutes.
5) Flip over and press for ten counts and cook for a minute or two.
6) Remove from pan, serve and enjoy.

Lunch Recipes

Cocktail of Prawns

Ingredients:
Tabasco sauce – optional
1 tbsp lemon juice
1 tbsp chives, chopped
¼ tsp paprika plus more
200g fat free Greek yogurt
150g cooked cocktail prawns

Directions:

1) In a small bowl whisk thoroughly the tabasco sauce (if using), paprika, chives, lemon juice and yogurt.
2) Place prawns in a medium bowl, pour in sauce and toss to mix.
3) Sprinkle with more paprika, best served if really cold.

Baked Salmon

Ingredients:
Freshly ground black pepper to taste
Salt to taste
1 tbsp lemon juice
One salmon fillet

Directions:

1) In an oven safe dish, grease with cooking spray and place salmon.
2) Rub on salmon freshly ground pepper, salt and lemon juice.
3) Pop in a preheated 350°F oven. Cook for 15 minutes or until middle of salmon is flaky.
4) Serve and enjoy.

Turkey Burger Cajun Style

Ingredients:

2 cloves garlic, chopped

1 green chilli, chopped – optional

1 tbsp Cajun spice mix

2 tbsps oat bran

1 egg

1.5 lbs lean turkey, minced

1 tbsp mustard – optional

1 tbsp ketchup – optional

Directions:

1) In a big bowl, mix garlic, chilli (if using), Cajun spice mix, and egg. Whisk well together for a minute.
2) Add minced turkey and mix with hands for a minute or two.
3) Add oat bran and mix again.
4) Shape into eight small burger patties.
5) Meanwhile, on medium fire, heat a medium nonstick frying pan greased with cooking spray.
6) Once heated, add patties and cook for 3 to 5 minutes per side.

7) Remove from pan and transfer to a serving plate.
8) Serve with a side of mustard and ketchup, if desired.

Vietnamese Beef

Ingredients:

10oz sirloin steak, cut into ½ inch cubes

¼ tsp vegetable oil

45g oyster sauce

2 tbsps soy sauce

1 tsp minced ginger

4 cloves garlic, crushed

Directions:

1) In a bowl, grate ginger. Mix in vegetable oyster sauce and soy sauce. Mix well.
2) Add beef cubes and marinate for an hour in the ref.
3) On high fire, place a nonstick skillet and heat oil. Add garlic and stir fry for a minute or until lightly browned.
4) Add beef and cook on medium fire for 10 minutes or until desired doneness is reached.
5) Remove from pan and serve.

Seafood Spanish Style

Ingredients:
Pepper and salt to taste
Half of a red chili, minced
1 tsp tomato puree
1 clove garlic, minced
1 packet of chilled pre-cooked seafood mix (squid, prawns, mussels)

Directions:

1) On medium high fire, place a medium nonstick fry pan and grease with cooking spray.
2) Once heated, add garlic and sauté for 2 to 3 minutes or until lightly browned.
3) Add seafood mix, cover and cook for 5 minutes or until water has evaporated fully.
4) Add tomato puree and mix well.
5) Season with pepper and salt to taste. Toss to mix well.
6) Cook for another minute.
7) Remove from pan, transfer to a serving plate, serve and enjoy.

Baked Mussels

Ingredients:

1 lb mussels

1 cup less fat cream cheese

¼ cup green onions, minced

1-inch long ginger, peeled

3 cloves garlic, minced

Directions:

1) In a bowl, mix cream cheese and green onions well. Set aside.
2) In a heavy bottomed pot placed on medium high fire, add mussels, garlic and ginger.
3) Cover and cook for 8 to 10 minutes or until most of the mussels have opened fully.
4) Turn off fire, uncover pot and let it cool for ten minutes.
5) One by one, remove the mussels and break off the empty shell and discard. Arrange shell with mussel on a baking sheet.
6) Meanwhile preheat oven to 350ºF.
7) Once all mussels are on the baking sheet, place cream cheese mixture on top of mussels. Ensure that you evenly place cream cheese

mixture on each mussel and cover it with the cream cheese mixture well.

8) Pop mussels in the oven and bake for 10 to 15 minutes or until cream cheese are melted and bubbly.

9) Remove from oven; let it rest for 5 minutes before serving.

Grilled Cod

Ingredients:

2 tbsps chopped green onions, white part only

1 lemon, juiced

¼ tsp ground black pepper

¼ tsp salt

½ tsp lemon pepper

1 tbsp Cajun seasoning

2 fillets of cod cut in half

Directions:

1) Prepare grill by preheating to medium high for around ten minutes. Grease grate with cooking spray.

2) Meanwhile, season cod fillets (front and back) with black pepper, salt, lemon pepper and Cajun seasoning.

3) Place on hot grill and cook for 3 minutes per side or until cod flakes easily. Ensure that you turn cod only once or else it may break into pieces.

4) Remove from grill, transfer to a serving plate and let it sit for 5 minutes.

5) Serve and enjoy.

Snack Recipes

Meringue

Ingredients:
1 cup of Truvia
½ tsp cream of tartar
4 egg whites

Directions:

1) Prepare egg whites and place at room temperature for an hour.
2) In a big bowl, whisked egg whites and cream of tartar until soft peaks form.
3) Slowly add sugar, one tablespoon at a time, while continuously whisking egg whites.
4) Preheat oven to 250ºF and grease a baking sheet with cooking spray.
5) Transfer egg whites into a piping bag and pipe icing onto prepared pan 1-inch apart.
6) Pop in the oven and bake until meringues are crisp and dry around 30 minutes.
7) Remove from oven, let it cool for 30 minutes before serving.

Oat Bran Muffin

Ingredients:
1 tbsp Truvia
1 tsp baking powder
6 tbsps zero fat yogurt
2 eggs
4 tsps reduced fat, no sugar added cocoa powder
6 tbsps oat bran

Directions:

1) Preheat oven to 350°F and line a muffin pan with muffin wrapper.
2) In a medium bowl, mix all dry ingredients together, except for Truvia.
3) In a small bowl, whisk eggs and yogurt until well incorporated.
4) Add truvia to the eggs and mix until dissolved.
5) Pour egg mixture into bowl of dry ingredients and whisk well to incorporate.
6) Evenly pour batter into 6 muffin lines. Pop into the oven and bake for 15 to 18 minutes or until cooked when toothpick is inserted in the middle no batter sticks to it.
7) Remove from oven, let it cool before serving.

Oat Bran Cookies

Ingredients:
2 tbsps skim milk
2 packets Splenda
2 tbsps Splenda brown sugar
1/8 tsp salt
¼ tsp baking soda
¾ cup oat bran

Directions:

1) Preheat oven to 375°F and grease baking sheet.
2) Blend Splenda, brown sugar, baking soda and oat bran in a food processor.
3) Pour into bowl and mix in milk. Whisk thoroughly.
4) Spray cooking spray on batter for a second. Mix well.
5) Spoon batter into baking sheet into 1 or 2 inch circles. Pop in the oven and bake for 6 minutes.
6) Remove from oven, let it cool and enjoy.

Ginger and Oat Bran Biscuits

Ingredients:
1 tbsp Truvia
1 ½ tsps dried ginger
1 ½ tbsps zero fat quark
3 tbsps oat bran
4 beaten egg whites

Directions:

1) In a medium bowl, mix well truvia, quark, oat bran, egg whites and ginger. The consistency of the batter should be thicker than a pancake.
2) On medium fire, place a nonstick skillet and grease with cooking spray.
3) Drop batter by spoonful around the skillet to create biscuit sized shapes.
4) Cook for 2-3 minutes per side or until desired brownness is reached.
5) You would need to cook all biscuits in batches and let it cool before storing in an air tight container.

Cappuccino Flavored Dukan Frappe

Ingredients:
16 ice cubes
4 tsps Truvia
1 cup cold skimmed milk
1 cup strong black coffee, cold

Directions:

1) In a blender, except for the ice cubes blend all ingredients together until foamy.
2) Add ice cubes and continue to blend until ice is crushed into small pieces.
3) Transfer to two serving glasses, serve and enjoy.

Fro-Yo

Ingredients:
3 tbsps boiling water
3 tsps strawberry flavored sugar free jelly
1 large tub of fat-free natural yogurt (500g)

Directions:

1) In a small bowl mix jelly and boiling water. Mix until jelly is totally dissolved. Set aside to cool for two minutes.
2) Then in a blender, blend jelly syrup and yogurt until smooth and creamy. Blend well so that jelly and yogurt are incorporated well in order to avoid jelly lumps once your yogurt ice cream freezes.
3) Once you are done blending the mixture thoroughly, place in a lidded container and freeze for 4 hours before serving.

Dinner Recipes

Meat Loaf

Ingredients:
1 tbsp garlic pepper seasoning
1 tbsp garlic salt
2 ½ tbsps chili powder
2 eggs
1 tbsp Worcestershire sauce
1 ½ pounds ground beef

Directions:

1) Preheat oven to 375°F and grease a loaf pan with cooking spray.
2) Mix eggs, Worcestershire sauce and ground beef in a large bowl.
3) Season with garlic pepper, garlic salt, and chili powder. Mix well again.
4) Place mixture into greased loaf pan and press to form a loaf.
5) Pop in the oven and bake for 35 minutes.
6) Remove from oven and let it stand for minutes before serving and slicing.

Grilled Lamb Chops

Ingredients:
2 lbs lamb chops
1 onion, sliced thinly
1 tbsp garlic minced
½ tsp black pepper
2 tsps salt
¼ cup distilled white vinegar

Directions:

1) In a re-sealable bag, mix onion, garlic, pepper, salt and vinegar. Seal the bag and shake until salt is dissolved.

2) Add lamb chops into the bag and marinate in the ref for at least two hours. While ensuring that you turn bag after an hour to ensure that all sides are marinated well.

3) On medium high fire, preheat grill and grease grate with cooking spray.

4) Remove lamb chops from bag and cover bony ends with foil. Place on the grate and grill for at least 3 minutes per side or until desired doneness is reached.

5) Remove from grill, transfer to plate, serve and enjoy.

Beef Kebabs

Ingredients:
¼ tsp thyme
1 bay leaf
¼ cup fresh lemon juice
2 tbsps Dijon mustard
¼ cup low sodium soy sauce
1 tbsp cider vinegar
14oz Beef fillet

Directions:

1) Cut beef into 1-inch cubes.
2) In a bowl, mix remaining ingredients thoroughly.
3) Add meat to seasoning mixture and marinade for at least two hours inside the ref. Ensure that you flip meat after an hour to marinate all sides of the meat.
4) Skewer the beef in Barbecue sticks and discard marinade.
5) Place kebabs in preheated grill on medium high fire and grill for 3 to 5 minutes per sie or until desired doneness.

6) Remove from grill, let it rest for 5 minutes before serving.

Chicken Curry

Ingredients:
½ tsp cayenne pepper
½ lemon, juiced
1 cup zero fat yogurt
1 tomato, sliced into wedges
2 skinless, boneless chicken breast halves, cut into ½-inch cubes
salt to taste
½ tsp truvia
½ tsp grated fresh ginger
1 bay leaf
1 tsp paprika
1 tsp ground cinnamon
3 tbsps curry powder
2 cloves garlic, minced
1 small onion, chopped
3 tbsps olive oil
½ cup water

Directions:

1) In a large nonstick sauce pan greased with cooking spray on medium high fire add onion and tomatoes.

2) Stir fry for 4 minutes or until lightly wilted. Add salt, truvia, ginger, bay leaf, paprika, cinnamon, curry powder and garlic. Stir fry for 2 minutes.
3) Add chicken breasts and stir fry for 5 minutes.
4) Add ½ cup of water, cover and cook for another 15 to 20 minutes.
5) Add yogurt, cook until heated through.
6) Remove from pan, serve and enjoy.

Roasted Rack of Lamb

Ingredients:

1 tbsp Dijon mustard

1 tsp black pepper

1 tsp salt

1 7-bone rack of lamb, trimmed and frenched

¼ tsp black pepper

1 tsp salt

2 tbsps chopped fresh rosemary

2 tbsps minced garlic

Directions:

1) Preheat oven to 450°F.
2) In a medium bowl, mix pepper, salt, rosemary and garlic. Add 1 tbsp water to wet ingredients and smear all around lamb rack.
3) On an oven proof nonstick skillet place on high fire, sear lamb for two minutes per side. Turn off fire.
4) Cover bony edges of lamb with foil and pop into the oven.
5) Cook for 12 to 18 minutes or until desired doneness.

6) Remove from oven and let it stand for 15 minutes before serving.

Tofu Stir Fry

Ingredients:
2 lbs firm tofu
1 tbsp tamari
1 lime
2 tsps minced fresh ginger root
2 tsps minced garlic

Directions:

1) On medium high fire, place a medium nonstick sauce pan and grease with cooking spray.
2) Stir fry ginger and garlic for two minutes.
3) Add tamari and tofu. Stir to mix.
4) Cover pan and lower fire to medium and cook for 20 to 30 minutes while ensuring to stir every 5 minutes.
5) Remove from pan and transfer to serving bowl.
6) Squeeze lime juice on top and serve.

Tandoori Chicken Fillets

Ingredients:
1-cm piece of peeled ginger
1 garlic clove
1 green chilli
1 lemon, juiced
2 tbsps zero fat yogurt
2 tbsps Tandoori Masala Spice mix
2 skinless chicken breast fillets

Directions:

1) In a food processor, blend ginger, garlic, green chili, lemon juice, yogurt and masala spice mix until smooth.
2) Score chicken two or three times per piece to allow flavors to seep in.
3) Place seasoning mixture into a bowl and add chicken. Toss well to mix. Cover with cling wrap and let it sit in the ref for a night.
4) Grill chicken for 6 to 8 minutes per side or until desired doneness is achieved.
5) Serve with a side of zero fat yogurt.

Conclusion

I hope that you have learned a lot about Dukan Diet and above all about the Attack Phase. With this book, you can start with the Dukan Diet plus the meal plan that I have readied above, you are ready to kick start your weight loss.

Printed in Great Britain
by Amazon

31507864R00033